IAN DAVIS

Can Swim!

The Official Guy's Guide to Pregnancy

THREE RIVERS PRESS
NEW YORK

Published by Three Rivers Press, New York, New York.
Member of the Crown Publishing Group, a division of Random House, Inc.
www.crownpublishing.com

THREE RIVERS PRESS and the Tugboat design are registered trademarks of Random House, Inc.

Originally published by Prima Publishing, Roseville, California, in 1999.

All products mentioned in this book are trademarks of their respective companies.

All characters and locations in this book are based on real persons and events, but in some cases, names have been omitted or changed to protect the privacy of the people involved. Therefore, any resemblance to actual persons, living or dead, or experiences is purely coincidental, unless authorized by the actual person mentioned.

Illustrations by Steve Skelton.

Printed in the United States of America

Library of Congress Cataloging-in-Publication Data
Davis, Ian.
My boys can swim! : a guy's guide to pregnancy. Ian Davis.
     p.   cm.
    1. Pregnancy, Popular works. 2. Pregnancy Humor. I. Title.
RG556.D29   1999
618.2'4—dc21
                        99-32679
                         CIP

ISBN 0-7615-2167-4

10 9
First Edition

To my wife, my daughter,
and the inventor of the epidural

Contents

INTRODUCTION • xi

1. The First Trimester (0 to 3 Months) • 1

Mission Impossible • 3

Health Insurance: Like a Good Neighbor
or a Bad Dream • 5

What's in a Name? • 7

C'mon Up Chuck • 14

Move Over Dolly Parton • 18

The World's Greatest Excuse • 20

2. The Second Trimester (4 to 6 Months) · 21

"Everyone's Getting Fat Like Mama Cass" · 23

Same Stadium, Different Playing Field · 25

No Pain, No Gain · 29

The OB/GOD · 29

Common Medical Tests · 30

Cop a Feel · 33

Sex Starved or Sex Kitten? · 34

Maternity Attire · 36

Blazing Saddles · 39

The Joy of "Regifting" · 40

3. The Third Trimester (7 Months to Delivery) · 43

Bankrupt Over Baby Stuff · 45

"Let's All Hold Hands and Sing 'Kumbaya'":
Those Dreaded Baby Classes · 49

In Search of Marcus Welby, M.D. · 54

The Invisible Man · 57

Baby Ex-Lax · 60

The Vital Signs · 60

Show Time! · 63

Check In/Check Out · 65

Mother Teresa · 68

Riding the Wave · 69

The Mother of All Shots: The Epidural · 70

The Only Day She'll Pray
to Be Constipated · 72

You Have to Go Through Hell
Before You Get to Heaven · 73

Where's My Reward? · 79

The Fun Begins! · 80

Things No One Tells You About
the Post-Delivery Experience · 83

Slice and Dice · 84

Final Words · 84

Epilogue · 87

ACKNOWLEDGMENTS · 91

Introduction

"HONEY, I'M PREGNANT." That you're reading this book means there is a good chance you've heard those earthshaking words, and that you share the excitement and sheer terror I felt when my wife Nada unleashed them on me a short time ago.

The memories are still vivid. There I was, lying in bed watching *Monday Night Football,* when Nada disappeared to take one of those early pregnancy tests. I grunted to myself, "purple strip—no way." We had begun trying just a few months earlier, and I wasn't quite ready to stop trying. When Nada returned to announce that the test was positive, my first reaction was "those tests are never accurate." But then she read

"99 percent accurate" off the label, and all of a sudden I felt like George Costanza when he finds out the woman he slept with is pregnant—"My boys can swim!" Next came a series of frightening thoughts: my beautiful sports car being bullied out of the garage by a big, ugly minivan; a crying baby on an airplane— and it's mine; horrific expenses; and enormous responsibility. My life as I knew it was over. My sphincter resoundingly clenched.

The next day I went to the bookstore seeking information and guidance. What did I find? Hundreds of books on pregnancy written for women. But nowhere to be found was a book to which a typical guy could relate. One that offered everything you *really* needed to know about the pregnancy experience and written with enough dripping sarcasm, humor, and irreverence to make it readable. I wanted to know about the daily growth of my wife, not the daily growth of the fetus. The fact that none existed led me to write this book. It's based on my experience with Nada, together with real-life anecdotes drawn from interviews with hundreds of other brave souls who survived the dramatic changes that will consume you and your wife for over nine straight months.

A few important disclaimers. First off, all pregnancies are different, so it's possible that your wife may be lucky enough to avoid some or even all of the more extreme behavioral changes discussed in this book. There are actually women who love being pregnant (hard to believe, but true). Second, I've tried to keep this book short enough to digest on a relatively brief domestic plane flight or within about four extended trips to the john. This is about all the time most guys will devote to reading about pregnancy. Therefore, don't expect comprehensive coverage of your wife's pregnancy experience here. If you need more information, consult her soon-to-be-created library on the subject, including the many parenting magazines she will subscribe to in the coming months. Finally, you should know that I know nothing about medicine. I cheated like hell in high school biology and still got a D. Anything that sounds even remotely like medical advice should be completely discounted. How's that for a fat legal disclaimer? My lawyer will be proud.

Since my wife Nada and I are the subject of commentary throughout the book, let me give you a quick lowdown on the two us: Nada is a vivacious, petite blonde whose personality is a cross between Bette Midler and Rosie O'Donnell. Her tell-it-like-it-is directness and her sense of humor were a big part of her success as a hairdresser (she's retired her scissors) to some of Washington, D.C.'s best-known personalities (she even did a year-long stint at the White House with Hillary). Not long after our daughter was born, a salesman in a clothing store asked Nada to describe what it really felt like to give birth. He had no idea who he was dealing with. "See that cash register over there?" she said. "Take that and shove it up your *#!@, and you'll catch the sensation." Without Nada's keen and often comedic insights about what women go through during pregnancy, I never could have written this book.

As for me, I'm your everyday Joe. Nothing too unique here. I'm a mid-thirties, quickly getting out of shape, pathetic golfer with a receding hairline (okay, I'm basically bald, but still in denial). My thinning hair, together with some gum recession, led my friend Ed to remark that my hairline and gums were having a race to the back of my head. I'm not sure what possessed me to spend so much time writing about the subject of pregnancy. More than once Nada found me in the kitchen typing away at 5:00 A.M., wondering, "Is he nuts? Writing a book about pregnancy? Gimme a break." I often had the same thoughts myself.

My Boys Can Swim!

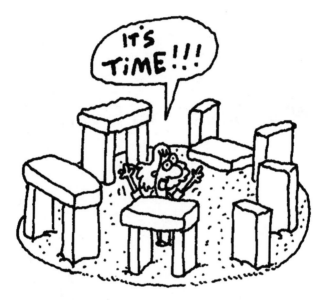

Recent studies indicate
Stonehenge was likely
a huge biological clock.

CHAPTER ONE

The First Trimester: (0 to 3 Months)

N ADA AND I *are at a hotel in Miami on vacation. A screaming infant on the flight down from Washington, D.C., has us both thinking the same thing: Is this parenting stuff for us?*

My sister-in-law, who lives near our hotel, visits us with her two kids. Her little boy asks me if I know Charlie. "Charlie who?" I respond. "Charlie Horse." With these words, his fist comes flying into my groin. For the first time in my life, I understand what seeing stars really means.

Later we visit some old friends with a newborn baby girl. They insist that I hold her. I immediately begin to sweat. The minute that baby hits my hands she starts crying uncontrollably. "She's always like that with strangers," they attempt to reassure me. But I know the truth. This kid senses that I am a klutz. She sees fear in my eyes. "Mommy, Daddy, this bald guy's gonna drop me. Let me go, loser!" is what those screams mean.

On our way back to the hotel, Nada announces that her biological clock is nearing expiration and that we should really start trying to have a baby.

Great timing. "Do you really think we're made out to be someone's parents?" I ask. "I can barely remember to floss daily."

"You'll be fine, honey. Just fine."

For some reason, I find this hard to believe.

If the idea of becoming a parent scares the hell out of you, you're not alone. This is one of life's few irreversible decisions. No refunds. No returns.

In my view, pregnancy *is* baby boot camp. There are some beautiful moments that strengthen the bonds between husband and wife. But there are also times you'll wonder if you're living in Superman's Bizarro World, where up is down, left is right, and logic is completely flipped on its head.

The first few months are easy. As the father-to-be, you'll live in pregnancy nirvana, basking in the glow of your impending fatherhood, and getting pats on the back from friends and family. "Congratulations! You finally did it!" There is no noticeable change in your wife's appearance or behavior just yet. Hey, this is great.

Then, like a sudden bolt of lightening, things change. The slight bulge in your wife's stomach hits you. Your mother-in-law is on the phone, quizzing you about job security. You're wandering aimlessly among feelings of denial, panic, and giddy excitement. One day, while you're sitting on the couch, telling yourself there's no way it's true, you suddenly find yourself wondering if there's lead paint in the spare bedroom and where to buy those outlet protector thingers. What the hell is going on?

Mission Impossible

BECAUSE nearly one in four pregnancies ends in miscarriage, spreading the news about your good fortune to a wide audience too quickly can be pretty risky. Since most guys are in a sheer state of denial anyway, it is not all that challenging to keep the secret under wraps for a good while. Getting your wife to do the same is another matter entirely.

If you do feel the urge to get the word out early, there are a number of credible reasons why it may be in your interest not to talk for, say, the full term of the pregnancy. First, once everybody knows there's a baby on the way, *your* life suddenly becomes insignificant, even in the eyes of your own family. Second, your phone begins ringing off the hook, with friends, family, and other well-wishers giving you the same startling and soon-to-be annoying salutation: "Hi Dad." After hearing this greeting for at least the 30th time, I mastered the technique of sounding amused and then quickly passing the phone to Nada. Finally, once you make an official public an-

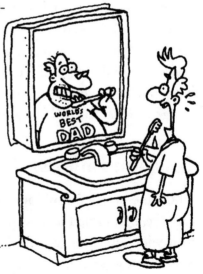

nouncement, every conversation for the next nine months will somehow lead back to the subject of pregnancy or child rearing. Unless you find the book *What to Expect When You're Expecting* a riveting tour de force, this situation may become just a bit overwhelming at times.

Health Insurance: Like a Good Neighbor or a Bad Dream

IF you're lucky, your health insurance will cover virtually all of the expenses related to the pregnancy and delivery. Mine didn't. I almost got sick when a friend told me the entire affair had cost him and his wife about $100. I was *far* less fortunate. If you haven't already done so, you may want to start quizzing your insurance company about what's covered and what's not.

Wondering just how high the tab for the medical bills will run? Try doing a little clandestine investigating of your doctor's personal spending habits. Any plans to build a summer home in the Hamptons? If so, you're basically screwed. How old are the kids?

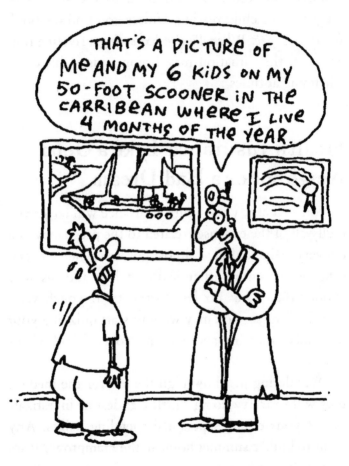

The First Trimester: (0 to 3 Months)

College age? Get ready to start writing some hefty checks.

What's in a Name?

UNLESS you're committed to naming your kid after Aunt Sarah or Uncle Ernie, you'll probably launch your search by consulting a book on baby names. As you scan the shelves of your local library or bookstore, you may be struck by the sheer number of books on the topic. Which one should you choose? No need to consult *Consumer Reports,* as I've done some exhaustive scientific research on this matter.

With all due respect to the true intellectuals who no doubt spent countless hours preparing these brilliant texts, they are *all the same.* I mean, how many different ways can you list "John" and "Mary"? Be especially wary of books that advertise themselves as being the "most comprehensive." They throw in every name ever used since the dawn of civilization, including my all-time favorite, "Odious" (Latin for "hateful"). Can you imagine? "He's so cute, let's name him Odious." Do you think *that's* ever happened? If you need a book to help in the search, do yourself a favor: Buy just one—*any* one.

Have you ever wondered why some parents actually bestow names on children that will inevitably cause them painful embarrassment during their formative years? I grew up around kids who had names like "Dick Byrd" and "Dick Bagg" (we referred to them as "Big Dick" and "Little Dick"). You probably have some good examples to add to this list.

The name "Dick" in particular seems to invite jokes, especially among heartless teenagers but also among adults at times. I remember the day I got a phone message from my former secretary asking me to return the call of Dick Itch. I figured it had to be a prank call from a friend, but my secretary was certain that this was a serious message. So for fun, I returned the call.

"Hello, I'm trying to reach Mr. Itch. Is he available?"

"One moment please. I'll connect you."

I couldn't believe it. How could anyone go through life with a name like Dick Itch? A momentary pause, then. . . .

"Dick Ditch speaking. How can I help you?"

Dick Ditch. Dick Itch. I wondered how many other people have made that mistake.

It seems like common sense not to give your kid a name that is easily mockable. Yet, to my amazement, people still do just that. My neighbor recently named his newborn "Thaddeus," which is Greek for "I'm a dork and should be beaten up."

Certain other names are so strongly associated with common stereotypes that they can influence both career paths and personalities. For example, Irving down the block is surely destined to be a tax lawyer sporting a bow tie, while Prescott is a banker with a passion for starched shirts and high-gloss shoe shines. It's also hard to warm up to a baby that's been given a name that you would normally associate with senior citizens. "This is baby Norman. Isn't he adorable?" Norman, of course, will be a moderately successful salesman of latex bras, with a preference for polyester over cotton. I find still other names just a bit too descriptive. Each time I meet someone named "Christian," I have the urge to say, "Well, hello Christian. I'm Jew." I mean, if "Hunter" is a legitimate name, why not "Archer" or "Rifleman"?

The people I really respect say, "Screw the past, I'm gonna make up my own name." Of course, this too can be a little risky. One mother fought for hours with my wife's OB about naming her kid "Vageena."

My friend Mike wanted to name his kid "Plummit" to mark what would happen to his income once the child was born.

The folks I feel the most compassion for have names from other cultures that just don't "translate" well into English. A college acquaintance from Thailand, Pissawatt, got hit pretty hard. Then there's that famous Chinese leader whose death kicked off the Tiananmen Square massacre, Hu Youbang (pronounced "who you bang"). Even my wife's name, Nada, which means "hope" in Croatian (her native land) always gets a big laugh in Miami. A brief vacation there led to nearly 100 "Deed ju know 'Nada' means nossing in espanish?" Just a bit annoying. My friend Jane, a Foreign Service Officer, told me that when she was stationed in Brazil she tried to convince a guy named Ignacio Phuck, who hailed from the village of Phuck (named after his family), to change his name because he'd have little luck selling his wares in the states with a name like that (I swear I'm not making this up). Ignacio, the president of Phuck Industries, was understandably proud of his name. Jane eventually issued him a visa with no name change. What the Phuck.

It's also tough to be named after a country or city. When first introduced to his new secretary, Rhodesia, my friend Todd responded, "wasn't your name changed to Zimbabwe?" (The fact that Rhodesia became Zimbabwe after independence clearly slipped by her, since her reaction to his comment yielded a pronounced "Say what?")

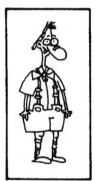

If you name your child 'LESTER' and he turns out like this, don't come crying to us.

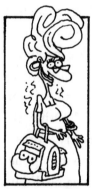

Most 'Hazel's are destined to live a life of cheap perfume and big purses.

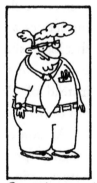

Most 'NORMAN's are a variation of this theme. (scientists are currently cross-checking samples of DNA.)

My real pet peeve when it comes to baby names has less to do with the actual choices than with the creative new-age spellings of traditional names. Just pick up any book on baby names and you'll see creative derivations of just about everything. It's no longer "Jackie," "Eric," and "Karen," but "Jacqui," "Eriq," and "Karyn." Now sometimes there *is* a reason for this. My friend Aerika, for example, is burdened with her mother's passion for Aerosmith. And what about names that are spelled in a way that doesn't even come close to how they're pronounced? How do the letters *p-h-o-e-b-e* become "Feeby"? Following this logic, shouldn't *phobia* really be pronounced *feebia*? To me, there is little advantage to being "Mikel" instead of "Michael." Other than annoying the hell out of people, is it really worth it?

As someone who has gone through life with a tough-to-pronounce name, I'd urge you to think twice before giving your kid a tongue-twister. The owner of my local Chinese restaurant, Mr. Han, loves to call his customers by their first names. "Howa you pronounsa your name?" he asked me during a visit. "Eee-In" I responded. He struggled for a while: "Yin, Alin. . . ." and then, "I got it. You mean lika Holiday Eeen."

Nada and I decided to name our first child (who we knew was a girl) after my Uncle Leonard. We struggled with "L" names for months on end. We finally settled on "Logan," which passed muster with our families but didn't go over very well with everyone else. "Why not 'Lauren' or 'Lisa'?" "That's a nice name, but what are you going to *call* her?" "Is that a family name?" I got so tired of people second-guessing us that I started responding to questions like "Why Logan?" by explaining that my family has a tradition of naming first children after major American airports. "We were torn between Kennedy, LaGuardia, and O'Hare, but finally settled on Logan." One humor-impaired person actually believed me.

Keeping the discussion of name choices strictly between you and your wife for as long as possible is something I highly recommend. You'll still get plenty of unsolicited, annoying input, but it will be nothing compared to what you'll get if you decide to ask for suggestions.

Why is it the rich and famous always find it necessary to give their children strikingly bizarre names? What are they trying to say to us? Here are a few hints.

STARS	KID'S NAME	MESSAGE
Bruce Willis/ Demi Moore	Rumer Glenn Scout Larue Tellulah Belle	We will do whatever it takes to get attention.
Frank Zappa	Dweezil Moon Unit	LSD is good.*
Eddie Van Halen	Wolfgang	What I wanted to name the band but my brother won the coin toss.
Sonny and Cher	Chastity	Anyone's guess.

*Ardent Zappa fans will forgive me here. I know Frank didn't do drugs, but you've gotta wonder with names like these.

C'mon Up Chuck

NOTHING quite signals the onset of a full-fledged pregnancy like a woman's first bout of morning sickness. If your wife experiences this common phenomenon, it will be by far the most uncomfortable and invasive physical aspect of the first stages of her pregnancy. I'm convinced the doctor who coined the phrase "morning sickness" was simply trying to trick women into thinking they'd feel better by the afternoon—and to trick their husbands into thinking they'd be safe by evening. No such luck. If your wife gets it, she'll feel like hell day and night. I remember my wife asking a friend how she would know if her vomiting is morning sickness or the flu? "If it's the flu, you'll get better," she responded.

Fortunately, not all women get morning sickness. If your wife is one of the unlucky ones, better go out and put some vomit bags in the glove compartment and toss a few more in her purse for good measure. Always be on watch for that "I'm about to get sick and it's your fault" look, which will appear just about every time she gets sick. Hey, she's got a point. It was your sperm that created this mess, after all.

I took Nada to dinner at the home of a prospective client, Señor Alberto Flores, a native of Argentina, during the height of a rather severe case of morning sickness. Nada was doing fine until Mrs. Flores began dishing out humongous plates of prime rib covered in gravy and ringed with fat. I was seated across from Nada at the table, watching intently as this hunk of rare meat was placed in front of her face. She was not pleased. This was in stark contrast with our host, who was seated next to her.

*"Mrs. Davis, we are delighted to have you here,"
said Señor Flores. The freaky thing was he looked and
spoke like Ricardo Montalban. I kept waiting for him to
say "rrrrrich Corinthian leather." "This beef is prepared
as we do it in my country. I know you'll enjoy it."*

*Nada was almost green. She had told me repeat-
edly she'd be fine at the dinner, as long as they didn't
serve beef. "I always wanted to try Argentine-style
beef, Señor Flores" she responded, as Señor Flores
gazed into her dish. "Mmmmm," she said, wrestling to
choke down her first small bit.*

*I thought she would yak on the spot. All I was
thinking about was how to escape what could quickly
become a diplomatic incident. I could see the headline:
"PREGNANT WOMAN STABS ARGENTINE
BUSINESSMAN; SHE DIDN'T WANT THE
BEEF." Fortunately, Nada made it through the
evening, meal intact, but I knew it would cost me later.*

If your wife has a bad case of morning sickness,
try to be as supportive as possible, although it's always
hard to come up with the right words. At first, you'll
feel compelled to be by her side while she does her
business. By the second month, her daily and late-
night yaks may become so commonplace that you'll

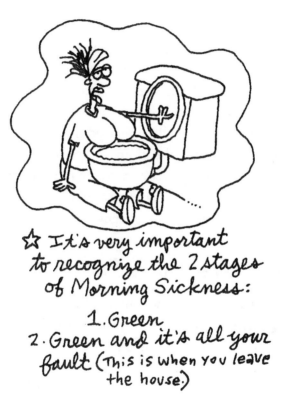

☆ It's very important
to recognize the 2 stages
of Morning Sickness:

1. Green
2. Green and it's all your
fault (This is when you leave
the house.)

hardly notice she's missing in action. The hardest part is when she calls out for help in the wee hours of the morning. I started out waking up with Nada and gently rubbing her back to show my concern. Because this affair became a nightly occurrence, my support gradually declined into yelling things from bed like "sounds like the dry heaves are almost over and you'll be back to bed soon, honey," to sleeping through the entire affair. She actually preferred the privacy.

Normally, after the third or fourth month, the nausea and vomiting associated with morning sickness shut off like a faucet. Pray your wife is lucky enough to avoid this aspect of pregnancy.

Move Over Dolly Parton

PERHAPS the most welcome physical change for many men and women during the initial stages of pregnancy is the amazingly rapid growth in most women's breasts—from modest to voluptuous in a matter of weeks. Other parts of a woman's body, like her hips and butt, will take a little longer to expand.

Be warned that some women's breasts may also develop what looks like an endless road map of blue veins, all leading to a series of bumps around the nipples that read, in Braille, "Don't even think about touching me." Her new and improved breasts are very likely to be highly sensitive to the touch, and they may even hurt. The pain does eventually go away. Unfortunately, so does the size.

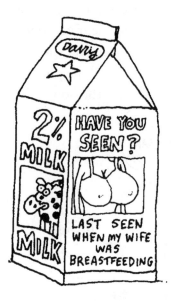

The World's Greatest Excuse

ONE of the best things about pregnancy is it provides the perfect excuse to gracefully bow out of any boring or undesirable social commitments. There are just an endless number of ways to use this pregnancy angle: "I'd love to come, but my wife's feeling kind of under the weather." "The doctor suggested that she stay off her feet." It's like magic. Everyone will completely understand, and may even feel sorry for you to boot. Meanwhile, you and your wife are off the hook. Guilt free.

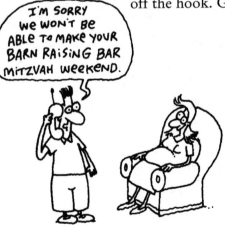

The First Trimester: (0 to 3 Months)

CHAPTER TWO

The Second Trimester: (4 to 6 Months)

"**W**elcome to Baby in Zee Sky. My name is Hannah. We have a huge zale toodaay."

"This woman's accent is getting on my nerves," I whisper to Nada. "I'll be back in a few minutes."

"Ve're clad you're beck," says Hannah as I return, taking me by the hand. "Your vife has exquisite taste. You vill luuuv vat she picked out."

"You're not going to like this," Nada warns me. "Nothing in this pile costs under $100 per piece."

She can't be serious. I mean, I know buying nice clothes will help lift her spirits after weeks of yakking her brains out, but these prices are ridiculous.

"Nada tells me how vunderful you've been wit ze

pregnancy. Not many men would let zere vives chop for zee clothes zey vant. I know you vant zee best for your pregnant wife, right?"

I hate this woman. She must have gone to the same school of guilt as my mother. Before I suggest to Nada that we leave, she pulls me aside.

"Listen," she says, "these clothes are a total ripoff. If I want high fashion, I'll wait till my fat ass gets back to normal. Let's get out of here."

The second trimester. This is when the action really begins and when the bucks start flying out of your wallet. Her fears of miscarriage have all but subsided, but say hello to a new set of fears that, together

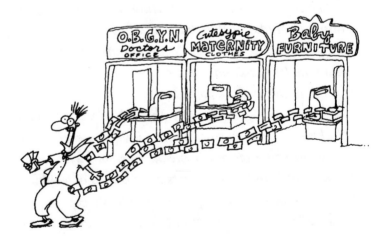

The Second Trimester: (4 to 6 Months)

with her physical discomfort and largeness, can alter your wife's behavior and greatly affect how your words and actions are perceived.

"Everyone's Getting Fat Like Mama Cass"

HAVING seen hundreds of pregnant women in your lifetime, you may feel pretty confident about what will happen to your wife's physical appearance now that she has a baby growing inside of her. I thought I did. Boy was I wrong. Even if you have seen a family member, or close friend, disrobed while fully pregnant or the famous Demi Moore photos in *Vanity Fair,* you *will* be shocked by how quickly and dramatically your wife's body can transform itself. Believe me, each day you witness this amazing metamorphosis you will acquire a new appreciation for having been born male.

This largeness in most cases is just part of the normal pregnancy process. Oftentimes, however, eating habits will be the determining factor between big and *really* big. Dave Barry, in his book, *Babies and Other Hazards of Sex,* notes that certain women develop absolutely voracious appetites during pregnancy and

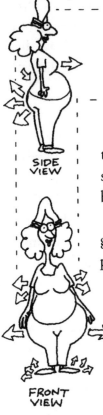

SIDE
VIEW

TOP
VIEW

FRONT
VIEW

attempt to jus-
tify this behav-
ior by pointing
out that they
are eating for
two. But what
these women need
to remember, Barry suggests, is that the
second one is the size of a Ping-Pong
ball, not Orson Welles.

If you're worried about your wife
gaining too much weight during the
pregnancy, don't sweat it. Fat and
happy is always better than thin and
cranky. Besides, most women lose the
weight gained during pregnancy
within six months after the birth.
Just let her be, and you'll save
yourself lots of heartache and possible
physical damage.

By the fifth month, the physical
changes you would expect to see—a more rotund
belly, larger breasts, and widening of the hip and butt
areas—will begin to show more prominently. Your

wife, who will probably be concerned, even obsessed, with her looks throughout the pregnancy, will at this point start asking you leading questions about her appearance: "You don't think I'm getting fat, do you?" "I feel so ugly. Do I look very different?" If you find her full-figured look more beautiful than ever before, as some men do, then by all means speak your mind. However, if that's not exactly the case, my advice in responding to her questions is to *lie through your teeth*. You will be forgiven. It's for a noble cause—her sanity and your safety. Yes, she'll know you're lying, but she'll give you huge credit for trying to be nice.

Of course, if there's more than one wide ass in the family, it's probably you. There must be some study out there that lays out all the reasons why men often gain weight along with their wives during pregnancy. Whatever the cause, watch out.

Same Stadium, Different Playing Field

EFFECTIVE communication between the sexes during a pregnancy versus before a pregnancy is like the difference between an undergraduate degree and a Ph.D. If you've read the book *Men Are from Mars, Women Are from Venus,* you have a head start, but consider yourself only moderately ready for pregnancy. Be prepared to marshal all of your best listening and interpretive skills. You will need them to translate a whole new language of subtle signs and turbulent emotions that emerges during the second trimester.

The Difference Pregnancy Makes in How Women See the World

CIRCUMSTANCE	PRE-PREGNANCY	DURING PREGNANCY
Your cologne:	"Smells so sexy."	"Makes me sick."
Her parting words as you leave to play golf:	"Have fun, honey."	"Have fun, bastard."
Visit by your mother:	"She's welcome any time."	"I hate her guts."

In my judgment, the root cause of these communication difficulties stems from the multiple fears and

It's not only important to
know what to say but also
what not to say and when
not to say it.

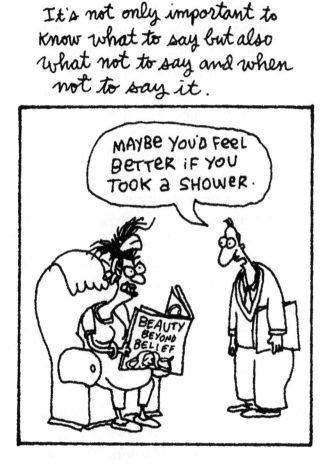

pressures a pregnant woman experiences, things that men just can't relate to very well—or at all. With the baby growing inside of her, she can never really escape the reality of impending parenthood. She worries constantly about everything—from something being wrong with the baby, to the biggest fear of all, labor and delivery. These fears often collide with some pretty energetic and unpredictable hormones.

My friend Chris told me his wife was so emotional about having a baby that she would sometimes cry after watching a Pampers or McDonald's commercial or reading a news story about a missing child. Chris's theory was that she would closely identify with the parents of the missing child and be overwhelmed by the sentimental beauty of a child celebrating a birthday with a Big Mac. Perhaps she just wanted a Big Mac.

Guys generally fear things that will happen *after* the child is born, like being a good financial provider, a role model, the future of their golf game, growing fond of cardigan sweaters, and not getting enough sleep. After all, nothing for us has really changed. Our bodies are pretty much the same. We go to work every day just like we did the year before. The bottom line is, the baby will not become a constant, ever-present source of concern and anxiety for you until the birth. It is this difference that lays the groundwork for possible misunderstandings.

No Pain, No Gain

SOME women never experience many of the uncomfortable symptoms associated with pregnancy (such as hemorrhoids, heartburn, aversion to certain odors, shortness of breath). They proceed through the entire deal as if nothing were all that unusual. If your wife does experience discomforts during her pregnancy, expect her friends and relatives to convey the familiar old wives' tale: Women who have difficult pregnancies often have easy deliveries. Now, call me stupid, but I think "easy delivery" is an oxymoron. How can passing a seven-pound object through a ten-centimeter hole be a walk in the park? You find me a woman that's had an easy delivery and I'll find you a man that enjoys having hemorrhoids.

The OB/GOD

DURING the second trimester you will hear more and more about your wife's obstetrician (OB). She will talk about this individual with great passion and intensity, almost like a teenager in heat. The OB is a pregnant woman's closest confidant, someone who has all the answers and the greatest degree of understanding. "He's the only man who really knows what I'm going through," she'll say. Of course, if your wife's OB is female, it's another story: "Only another woman can understand what I'm going through." Hence, the name "OB/GOD."

Regardless of how kind and thoughtful you may be during the pregnancy, this Zen-like figure will make you look like an uninformed, insensitive twit. You will marvel at the time your wife takes to primp herself prior to a visit with the OB/GOD, even though she hasn't put on a stitch of makeup for you in months.

Common Medical Tests

TWO common tests unique to pregnancy are the amniocentesis (or "amnio" in pregnancy lingo) and the sonogram. Both are typically given during the second trimester.

Just a Pinprick

The amniocentesis tests the genetic health of the fetus. If your wife elects to take this test, get ready for a dramatic, high-anxiety experience. Also be prepared to write a big check, because it ain't cheap and some health insurance plans do not cover its cost. The procedure involves sticking the mother of all needles—seven inches long—into the mother's belly and through the uterus in order to extract fluid from the amniotic sack. If your wife, who will probably not want to look, asks you if the needle is as big as her friends described it, make sure to at least try to play it

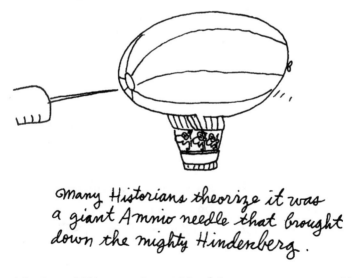

Many Historians theorize it was a giant Amnio needle that brought down the mighty Hindenberg.

cool. Do not remark, like my friend Chris did, "It's the biggest damn needle I've ever seen!" His wife had to come back on another day to do the test. In fact, if you hate getting shots and can't stomach watching someone else getting one, *do not* watch this procedure. Once the needle is in position, it takes some time before the full load of amniotic fluid is withdrawn. It's not a pretty sight.

Lost in Space

Sonograms are a lot more fun than the amnio, especially when you get your first glimpses of the baby. Your wife will want a sonogram done at nearly every doctor visit, which is fine as long as you've got decent health insurance or lots of cash, because it ain't cheap either.

Each time your wife has a sonogram, you'll get a nice black-and-white photo to keep as a memento. While you and your wife may find this picture highly significant and display it proudly to family and friends, be assured that everyone else will think you're giving them a Rorschach test. The still photo just doesn't capture the moment very well, and will often make the fetus look like a Klingon warrior. Still, you'll find yourself saying things like "Isn't this amazing?" while pointing to the picture of your alien child.

My first sonogram experience was extremely disappointing. As I peered into the monitor, I kept looking for some sign of life, but all I saw was faint movement in a smoky-like galaxy. The doctor was saying, "Now here's the head, the feet, hands. . . ." *Where? What? I can't see a thing!* I learned later on that my wife's first sonogram took place just a bit too early for the untrained eye to pick up much, so I stopped feeling so dumb.

Cop a Feel

As soon as your wife begins to show in a big way, you may wonder if someone secretly sewed a bull's eye on her belly that reads, "Please rub me." There seems to be this weird bond among women when it comes to pregnancy, and the belly rub is the unspoken show of kinship. Nada became obsessed with rubbing her own belly and with wanting everyone to touch it. She also liked to freak out my single friends by exposing her belly and asking them to rub it. "This is what you have to look forward to," she would say to my dedicated-bachelor friend Ed. Each time Ed saw her belly, he thanked the lord for birth control.

Sex Starved or Sex Kitten?

As the more intrusive physical and emotional symptoms of pregnancy begin to kick in, you start to wonder what will become of your sex life. Let's cut to the chase. Some women love sex when they are pregnant. Others would prefer spending their pregnancy locked in a room with your mother. Of course, these are the two extremes, and most women fall somewhere in the middle. My friend Dave told me that he and his wife actually had sex *more* often during the time she was pregnant than before. I hate to break it to you, but your chances of being like Dave are sort of like leaving the porch light on for Jimmy Hoffa. I hope you get so lucky, but don't count on it.

Probably the biggest concern most men and women have about sex during pregnancy is hurting the baby. This fear becomes especially poignant when you start to feel the baby move. I kept picturing my child bobbing and weaving inside the uterus in an effort to avoid getting poked. If your wife believes you might hurt the baby during intercourse, then welcome to the world of celibacy. Your only hope is to ask her OB/GOD to convince her she has nothing to worry about. According to several doctors I spoke with, intercourse is generally safe during pregnancy. However, there have been cases involving particularly well-endowed men penetrating a little too far and causing problems associated with high-risk pregnancies. Most of us, however, whether we want to believe it or not, do not fall into this superhuman category, so we have little to worry about.

Intercourse becomes especially challenging during the final few months. Her girth will make traditional missionary-style sex all but impossible for you and uncomfortable for her. Your best bet, if you're still in the game, is

THIS IS THE ONLY POSITION THAT'S WORKING FOR US RIGHT NOW!

to experiment with different positions. I'm told there are some that work well, although I can't speak from experience. I was temporarily sidelined for the duration of the pregnancy at right about the seventh month.

Maternity Attire

ONE thing you and your wife will quickly discover about maternity clothing stores is that they are all owned and managed by the same sophisticated Mafia syndicate that controls the sale of diamonds and wedding dresses. I'm convinced an annual meeting of the Maternity Clothing Producers Cartel (MCPC) takes place wherein an agreement is reached to keep prices on fashionable maternity clothes at exorbitant levels. The cheap stuff is put out just so women will be forced to make the choice between looking like a dowdy farm girl ("I couldn't be seen in that" is the intended reaction) or a hip, pregnant chick.

Many women regard maternity clothes as nothing less than humiliating. Nada is convinced that the big collars, bows, and puffy sleeves so common to maternity wear are supposed to balance out the big butt and engorged stomach. "They make you look like an overgrown five-year-old. Slap some cotton candy in your hand and you're ready for the World's Fair."

Each time Nada ventured into MCPC members' quarters, I warned her to view the sales help with great suspicion ("pawns of the Mafia kingpin"). I just can't believe that some clever entrepreneur hasn't come up with an attractive and affordable line of pregnancy attire. Maybe someone tried, but he or she is at the bottom of the Atlantic Ocean in cement shoes.

One key part of the maternity wardrobe that most

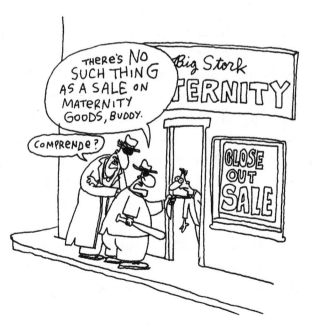

men find startling is maternity underwear. You've probably never seen this stuff (why would you have?), so brace yourself: These parachute-like undies are big enough to fit an NFL defensive lineman. Of course, some lingerie stores carry a more attractive lace version but at an astronomical cost (about $20 a pair). So don't be shocked if one day your wife disrobes and she is wearing a Glad Bag seemingly pulled up to her chin. She may even be wearing your underwear, which may be both more comfortable and certainly more attractive, than the parachutes.

Another critical component of maternity wear is shoes. About midway through the pregnancy, Nada complained that none of her shoes would fit. Now, I'd heard about women's feet swelling—and even growing half an inch or more—during pregnancy, but I always suspected that this was just a devious gimmick dreamed up by Nordstrom's to encourage women to purchase new shoes. So for fun, I took out a ruler and measured Nada's feet, and—damn, they had grown about half an inch.

In fact, close to 80 percent of pregnant women actually go up one-half shoe size during the second to third trimester, and the change is usually permanent.

Could somebody please explain to me why this happens? It's obvious why breasts grow larger and hips wider, but feet getting longer? Is it a balance thing? Please write to me if you figure this out.

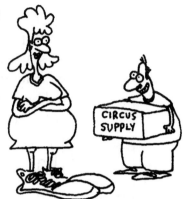

Blazing Saddles

I DIDN'T know whether to laugh or cry when my colleague, who was eight months pregnant at the time, delivered a fart that about knocked me out of my chair during a presentation meeting with a key client. She was so embarrassed I thought she'd give birth right there on the spot. Soon after this incident I learned that women experience an extraordinary amount of gas during pregnancy and that they often cannot control its release.

The information is intended to prepare you for the hillbilly opera you may experience during your wife's pregnancy. Most couples who have been through a pregnancy will be very forgiving if your wife happens to fart or burp in their presence. Your single friends, or those without kids, may just chuckle. Whatever the reaction, be assured that your wife will be mortified, at least initially, if she happens to

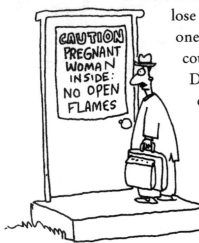

lose control in front of anyone but you. Unless, of course, she's like my friend Deborah, who loved to exhibit her new farting prowess at public events ("Hey guys, listen to this. . . ."). In this case, it was her husband who was mortified.

The Joy of "Regifting"

DON'T underestimate the benefits of a baby shower. It's one of the major bonuses of the pregnancy experience. Not only do friends and family load you up with all kinds of useful (and expensive-to-buy) baby goods, but you usually end up with extra stuff or duplicates that you can unload as gifts at others' baby showers. Hence, the joy of what I call "regifting."

The abundance of stuff you'll receive opens up the possibility of multiple regiftings. We passed on one gift we received at Nada's shower to a friend who was a bit short on cash. He then re-regifted it to his boss's wife at her shower. My question is, will the recipient of the re-regifted gift regift it yet again? I guess I'll never know.

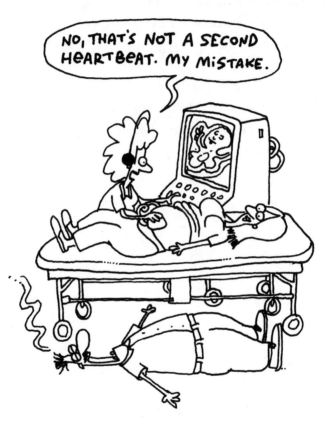

CHAPTER THREE

The Third Trimester: (7 Months to Delivery)

THE DELIVERY ROOM *is bright and filled with shiny metallic equipment. Dr. Newman announces that it's time for the final push. It has been nearly two hours since Nada's heavy labor began and since I first had the urge to go to the bathroom. I've been holding it in all this time so as not to miss the big moment. Now I'm doing that funny little dance to protect my bladder from imploding. The nurse thinks I'm demonstrating my excitement over becoming a dad. "Stay focused," I keep telling myself.*

"There it is. I see the head," says Dr. Newman. "Just push, one more time."

My beautiful daughter emerges.

"Hold it a second. Nurse Thomas, we're getting a funny reading here. . . . Why, I . . . think . . . you're going to have triplets!"

I about pee in my pants. "But, but, what about the sonogram, and the. . . ." Before I can spit it all out, three crying babies are in front of me.

"The lord works in mysterious ways," Nurse Thomas says to me.

I can't respond. All I can think of is what I did to piss him off. I see a flash of light.

"Honey, wake up. You're having a bad dream," I hear Nada say.

"No, it was a nightmare."

By the seventh month you will have almost forgotten what it was like before your wife became pregnant. People will begin asking her, "Haven't you had that baby yet?" This is guaranteed to ruin her day. Even you may wonder just how much larger she can grow. While you and your wife have entered the home stretch, these last few months are by far the longest and most trying of the entire deal. If you survived the first six months with few problems, more power to you. Don't expect such smooth sailing as you head closer and closer to D-Day.

Shopping sprees for baby stuff will likely commence around this period. Once you've crossed the eight-month threshold, your wife has entered what I call the "I can't" phase of the pregnancy ("I can't breathe, I can't walk, I can't go to the bathroom, I can't sleep, I can't eat," and so on). And of course, you're close to where the rubber hits the road—labor and delivery.

Bankrupt Over Baby Stuff

SOME of the best advice I received when Nada first got pregnant was from my friend Hank: "Don't get sucked into buying all that baby stuff," he said. Hank and his wife gave birth in China, and they survived just fine with basic baby supplies, including a folding card table (changing table), cardboard box (crib), and regular off-the-shelf bottles, nipples, and pacifiers. "Be careful about merchants of baby stuff," Hank warned. "Before you know it, they'll have you convinced you need double or triple what's really necessary." Boy, was he right.

The first time you enter one of those gigantic baby megastores stores you feel like you're in the middle of Japan with only a phrase book. Everything looks familiar, but you have no idea how to communicate what you want or even where to begin.

Nada and I decided to seek guidance at the customer counter during our first visit. "Here's what *we* recommend for the basics," the representative kindly informed us. It was then that I learned the first word unique to pregnancy, the *layette.* That's French for "You must buy at least one of everything in this store." The layette is actually a lengthy list of baby stuff designed for ignorant first timers like you and me.

We started with baby bottles and pacifiers. Easy, right? Wrong. This baby megastore had around thirty different versions in assorted shapes, colors, and sizes. Which one do you choose? I returned to customer service to get some advice. "James to baby bottles for customer assistance." When I met James, who appeared to be about 17 years old, I wondered what advice he would be able to impart, since I had to assume he had few, if any, children. I guess I'm a pretty good judge of character, given the substance of our conversation.

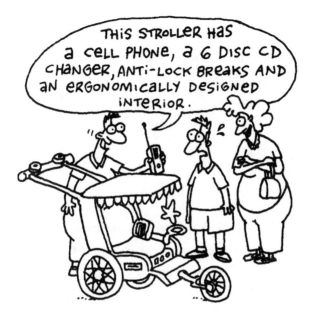

"How can I help you folks?" James asked.

"Well, we need some help selecting a baby bottle. There are just so many to choose from, and they all seem about the same" Nada began.

"Well," James responded, "let's see. These bottles have tilted heads. These are the most narrow. This one has the widest mouth and a handle in the middle, while this bottle can hold the most liquid. . . ."

I was awestruck by these profound insights. "But

do they operate much differently from one another?,"
I queried.

"Dude, they're all pretty much the same. The only real difference is price."

He was clueless but honest. "Any particular one you would recommend?" I asked.

"Yeah, the Nuk."

"Why?"

"Cool name."

It seemed to me that decisions on just about everything—the baby carriage, car seat, crib, changing table, even diapers—were made more difficult by the gross excesses of choices offered by those colossal baby megastores. I'm sure our parents had it much easier. They probably were able to purchase baby stuff like generic commodities at the local drug store: "We'll take eight bottles, a baby carriage, and a crib, thank you." No debating colors, features, or models. It was the Henry Ford approach: our color choices are black and black. If you're like me, you will long for these simpler days of baby shopping.

You will need to get the must-have baby things. A quick check with your wife's female friends or with family members with kids can really help you overcome the initial ignorance we all feel when shopping for baby gear for the first time. But be careful. On selections of simple, inexpensive items like bottles and pacifiers, you're in safe territory. However, for bigger ticket items like cribs and carriages, hold on to your wallet. These necessities can range in price from $50 to $1,000, depending on the brand and the store.

One more thing: If you decide not to accompany your wife on this baby stuff treasure hunt, as most men do, don't go complaining about the credit card bill. In either case, you will be amazed at how much all this stuff will cost you.

"Let's All Hold Hands and Sing 'Kumbaya'": Those Dreaded Baby Classes

WHEN you find yourself checking into birthing classes, you know you've made it into the home stretch. While I've yet to meet a man who actually enjoys attending these sessions, they do force you to realize that you really will become a father very soon. The classes also serve as training camp for the big day.

One of the first things you will realize, whether

you're taking the so-called Lamaze or general baby-care classes, is that most of your male brethren dread being in the class as much as you do. By the way, have you ever wondered who or what the hell Lamaze is anyway? I've heard varying stories, but have come to the conclusion that "Lamaze" is just some fancy French word that doesn't mean much of anything, sort of like what Häagen Dazs is to ice cream. If the class was called "Coping with the Excruciating Pains of Childbirth," who would go? But who can resist the exotic European insights of the "Lamaze?" Brilliant marketing, wouldn't you say?

Unlike our fathers' generation, where attending classes like these was seen as wimpy, you will have no choice. Neither will your compatriots. As such, you will quickly find yourself bonding with the other guys in the class, sharing stories about your wives, how bored you are, and complaining about the person who keeps asking a stream of stupid questions. (One woman in my class actually asked "Should you save the umbilical cord after it dries up?" I wondered, what the hell do you do with a dried umbilical cord? Mount it on a display? Show it to your friends at parties? "Hey Steve, bet you can't guess what this is. Catch!")

I really can't recall learning anything particularly

useful during these classes. Nada and I took Lamaze and general-baby care. You seem to spend a lot of time receiving extensive training on breathing techniques designed to help ease the pain during contractions. Now that I've witnessed firsthand a labor and delivery, I can tell you from experience that these breathing techniques have little or no value when your wife is suffering real-life contractions. Just imagine someone kicking you in the balls every couple of minutes, which I imagine is how labor pains would feel for men. Would your spouse asking you to breathe deeply while counting to ten really ease your suffering?

Women in labor usually start out trying to use the breathing exercises; some end up resorting to desperate prayers that the pain will just go away soon or urgent pleas for drugs. In any case, you will be forced to endure these lengthy breathing exercises, which your wife may insist that you continue even in the comfort of your own home.

The most dramatic moment of the Lamaze class is watching the film that shows a real-life delivery, in graphic detail. I'd seen *flashes* of films like this one on the Learning Channel (TLC), but always had my handy remote control in hand to quickly change the station. But now you're trapped. The version we saw featured an overweight couple in their mid-thirties from the Bronx. They were not completely unattractive, but the thought of watching John Belushi and Roseanne look-alikes go through labor and delivery together was less than appealing. Now, keep in mind, what you see on TLC are "highlight" films. Clever TV executives know that no guy in his right mind would be interested in viewing multiple scenes of a woman in deep labor moving from a shower, back to bed, sitting doggy style—all the while groaning in agony. In class,

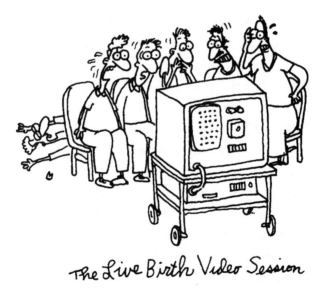

The Live Birth Video Session

you get to see it all. The full monty. And as you watch this horror show, consider whether you would rather sit through the rest of it or get root canal surgery. I guarantee this will be a tough choice. "So, what did you all think?" our enthusiastic instructor asked when the hour-long film from hell came to an end. For the first time since the class started, there was dead silence (even from Mrs. Dried Umbilical Cord).

Instructors for pregnancy-related courses are a special breed. They share an unusual passion for the subject matter, so much so that a seemingly simple question can generate excruciatingly detailed and lengthy responses that either annoy you or put you to sleep. Watch out for instructors who have never given birth themselves. They typically display cult-like attributes, such as glazed eyes and an exceptionally calm demeanor, when talking about the labor and delivery. Nada and I grew to like our teacher (despite her annoying habit of ending every sentence with "mmmkay"). Her soothing voice and detailed explanations worked on me like Sominex. At one point, as she was explaining how to bathe the baby ("Gently rub the sponge over the scalp, *mmmkay*. Softly caress her hands, *mmmkay*."), I nodded off, only to be awakened by a sharp elbow in my rib cage. Probably the most memorable moment of my classroom experience occurred when one woman suggested that we invite in a guest speaker from academia. Her astute husband responded, "Where's Macadamia?"

One other thing you may find annoying about these classes was constantly being referred to as "coach." My feeling was that I hired a medical doctor to be the coach, and that I was more like an enthusiastic fan trying to encourage my star player to hit a home run. Moreover, once you're in that delivery room, do you think your advice as "coach" has any real credibility? "Just shut up and get me the doctor" is what you'll likely hear if you try to demonstrate your newfound medical knowledge. Your best bet is to leave the advice business to the professionals.

In Search of Marcus Welby, M.D.

BECAUSE you will need a pediatrician to come to the hospital to examine your newborn and to care for the baby after the birth, it's important to spend some time interviewing candidates for the job. You must feel comfortable with and confident in your baby's pediatrician, so choose one carefully. Here's a list of interview questions to help you with your search. The answers will reveal just about all you will need to know to make a wise decision.

1. "Can you name three words that rhyme with *Kwanza*?" This will test the pediatrician's credentials and intelligence (hint: Lufthansa, George Costanza).

2. "If I call you at home repeatedly at 3 A.M. to inquire about my baby's sleeping habits, will that piss you off?" This will test for patience and accessibility.

3. "I've always wondered why we refer to an airplane pilot's domain as a *cockpit.* Any thoughts on that?" This should reveal if they have any sense of humor, a much needed commodity when dealing with a newborn baby.

An acquaintance of Nada's recommended a pediatrician who was covered under our insurance plan. We decided to make an appointment for an interview. A bit nervous and anxious, we were called from the waiting room for our meeting.

"Well, hello. I'm Dr. X." (The name has been deleted to protect the innocent.)

For the first time in my life, I came face to face with Pat, the androgynous person from Saturday Night Live. *I had neglected to ask Nada if the pediatrician was male or female. From the look on Nada's face, she had no clue.*

"So, what can I tell you about myself?" he, I mean she, asked.

"Well you can start by . . . ," I couldn't bring myself to ask. I looked to Nada to raise the first question. She, too, was at a loss for words. I decided to kick things off. "So, you take care of babies?" A brilliant start.

"Yes, that's what pediatricians do."

"And you seem to have a thriving practice."

"We do okay."

I just couldn't go on. Only one thought was racing through my head: How the hell we ended up in the office of Dr. RuPaul. It was time for a quick exit.

"This has been extremely helpful," I said. "Thank you for your time. We'll be in touch soon."

Another doctor we interviewed had a terrible case of what William Safire once called "upspeak." That is, making statements in the form of a question. "My name is Dr. Ryan? Thank you for dropping by? I'm happy to answer any questions you have?" It was like an ongoing game of *Jeopardy*. The interview didn't last long either—we were out of there in less than fifteen minutes?

The Invisible Man

As you and your wife inch closer to the fateful due date, you may need to learn how to cope with her steady stream of legitimate complaints about this or that ailment and endure her endless criticism of your good fortune for having been born male. You may even discover what I like to call "It's all about me and the baby" syndrome. Your problems? Who cares. Face it: In her view, whatever you're dealing with is nothing compared to what she's going through during these last few months of pregnancy. Begin to count the number of times you are told "Men have it so easy" or (as one of Nada's friends more delicately put it) "Men suck." Your wife's girlfriends, especially those with children, will probably reinforce this view that men got the luck of the draw. So don't go complaining to them about your wife's behavior. You'll get no sympathy there.

The "I can't" phase referenced earlier is something that the typical pregnant woman experiences toward the end of the third trimester, and for good reason. The baby has grown so large inside of her that there's not much room left in there for her vital organs, which are being pressed to the limit. Discomforts are common, even when the baby is in an ideal position for liftoff. She may find that a decent night's sleep is a fantasy, a normal bowel movement a dream, a casual walk through the mall a struggle. Her extraordinary girth may force her to regularly sit in a position you may consider rather unladylike: legs spread and her belly falling down in between. This is no reflection on her social graces. It's just about the only way she'll feel comfortable.

You may also discover that you've taken a backseat in bed—to your wife's pillow. Stuffed between her legs or under her belly, it may be just about the only thing that eases her discomforts and helps her sleep. It will also form a natural barricade in case you start thinking about pursuing any late-night action.

Nothing about this "I can't" phase will put your wife in a good mood. On the contrary, be on special guard during this phase, as you may find it increasingly difficult to do anything right. Also, your wife may be so on edge that she has the potential to take out her aggressions on total strangers. Nada nearly assaulted a meter maid for giving us a parking ticket.

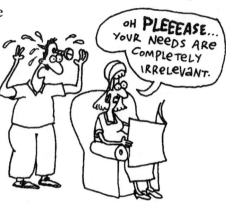

And don't be surprised if you start learning more from the wisdom of the "they" people. You know, "They don't recommend that hospital anymore" and "They say minivans are a must-have for kids." You will never win an argument with "they" no matter what facts you bring to the table. "They" always know best. I thought my grandmother had a special in with the "they" people since she talked about "they" and "them" in reference to every decision I've ever made in my life. I once pressed her to the wall on the origin of some "they" info. "I heard it on a Maxwell House commercial," she said. Well, okay then, it must be accurate.

Baby Ex-Lax

As your wife's discomforts reach a peak during these final few weeks of pregnancy, she may become vulnerable to accepting any prescription, however crazy, to expedite the birth. Some common antidotes include drinking red raspberry leaf tea, eating spicy foods, taking car rides along bumpy roads, and even having more sex. During our Lamaze class, one woman asked under what circumstances can sex at the end of the pregnancy bring on labor? I wanted to say, "When the sex is between your husband and another woman."

Because Nada had a difficult pregnancy, growing to enormous proportions weeks before her due date, she tried just about every wacko remedy to "get this @#*! kid out of me" (a near-exact quote). Of course, nothing worked and she ended up delivering our baby on her exact due date.

The Vital Signs

A WEEK prior to the due date is when you enter the drop zone. My biggest fear by this time was not the birth but that Nada's water might break inside my beautiful new car. Some women can gush literally gallons of water without warning, so you may want to place water-resistant materials over those things you cherish that may be visited by your wife's derriere. Also, if you have a dog, keep it away from your wife when her water breaks. My friend's Labrador Retriever thought the water was some kind of treat and began licking it off the floor.

At this stage, the pregnant woman often embarks on a frenetic cleaning and reorganization regimen. Commonly known as "nesting," this is a period of tremendous velocity with little direction. You'll look around your house and see nothing that really needs to get done. She'll see East Beirut. Failure to cooperate if

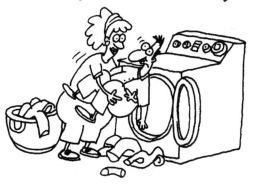

During the Nesting Period, it's best to stay clear of the washing machine.

and/or when she enters nesting mode can often lead to dire consequences. It's best just to hop on the bandwagon when it's headed your way.

By this time, you should have the stuff you'll need for the hospital all packed up and ready to go in advance. Plan for two nights, just in case. Among various other essentials, don't forget these three critical necessities:

1. *Food*. An airplane meal is gourmet dining compared to hospital food. One popular meal at my hospital was Salisbury steak. Didn't they stop making this stuff when TV dinners became obsolete? What moron picked this menu? I can almost picture the cafeteria planning session. "After all these women have been through," said cafeteria lady #1, "we ought to give them a truly nutritious, tasty meal, like Salisbury steak." "Yes!" responded cafeteria lady #2, "a great choice. They'll love it."

2. *A sleeping bag*. If you have to stay overnight, a sleeping bag will be far more comfortable than the so-called "beds" provided for fathers. Trust me, you won't want to spend the night on one of these medieval torture instruments. I'm convinced these

sleeping implements were chosen by female nurses in an effort to inflict an equal amount of back pain on expectant husbands as their labor-stricken wives.

3. A $100 bill. Keep it handy, just in case the anesthesiologist is reluctant to give in to your wife's pleas for an epidural.

Show Time!

MY friend Jessica was on the phone with Bill, her boss, when she went into labor. Her contractions were strong, and she felt it was time to head to the hospital.

"Umm . . . Bill," she interrupted him midsentence. "I've gotta hang up like right now. I'm in labor and I think it's time!"

"Cindeeeey!" Bill screamed out to his own wife. "Jessica's on the phone and she's in labor. Any suggestions on what I should do?"

"Yeah," Cindy responded. "Hang up."

When your doctor gives you the Bob Barker "Come on down" line, he or she may also suggest that your wife hop in the shower before heading for the hospital. First-time deliveries are usually long, drawn-out affairs, leaving plenty of time at this point for a quick shower. This could very well be the only chance your wife has to bathe herself for the next few days. Some women opt to shower, whereas others are feeling too much pain or anxiety to consider anything but getting to the hospital. Either way, *your* greatest concern will be getting the hell out the door as quickly as possible.

If your wife decides to take the shower route, don't expect her to bypass the regular makeup application and blow-dry treatment. After all, she's about to have a critical encounter with the OB/GOD. She's got to look good. When I found Nada, in mid-contraction, primping herself for the journey, I began to wonder, "are we going to a black-tie affair or a birth?"

My friend Bill told me that his wife gave birth to their second child in the back seat of their car on the highway. Labor and delivery for their first child had taken nearly twenty-four hours. When the doctor told them to come in, they headed down the highway thinking they had plenty of time, only to be stopped by a combination of rush-hour traffic and a major accident. Suddenly, voilà, the baby's head started to emerge. To their credit, the backseat delivery was a success.

You have probably heard other stories of couples with backseat babies. You may even be having nightmares about delivering your child without professional help. *It can happen!* My extreme paranoia led me to test drive the route to the hospital multiple times in preparation for the big day. I also consulted with the AAA on possible shortcuts and took the car in for an inspection. I was taking no chances.

A woman's sense of urgency about getting to the hospital is enhanced by the discomfort of the ride. Sitting upright in a car while in labor is uncomfortable enough for her. Add in a few bumps and potholes, a swerve here, a sudden stop there, and what she's feeling is a cross between Disney's Space Mountain and the annual sale at Filene's Basement.

Check In/Check Out

I STRONGLY encourage you to tour your hospital's birthing center prior to the delivery. If you're expecting to find something akin to the bedlam you see during episodes of ER—doctors yelling, women screaming in pain, doors flying open unexpectedly—

you're in for a big surprise. These places can be almost serene. Doctors walk calmly in and out of rooms. You'll wonder, "Hey, where's all the action?" You won't realize till later that this environment is part of an overall plan to keep expectant parents calm and slightly off balance. "All of our rooms are equipped with TVs and VCRs for your relaxation," our tour guide kindly informed us. Relaxation? I could just picture it. "Honey, would you mind if I flick on the Redskins-Giants game while you sit there in agony? I mean, why should we both suffer?" While there may be a calming quiet within the public areas of your birthing center, believe me, behind closed doors there's hell to pay.

It's a good idea to get the registration stuff as much out of the way as possible prior to arriving at the hospital. This will lessen your time with the registration clerk responsible for admitting your wife to the birthing center. I can assure you this individual will share none of your excitement or sense of urgency about getting your wife to the delivery room. He or she will run you through a laundry list of requests for mundane information (insurance plan, Social Security number, etc.) while your wife sits nearby suffering. To the clerk, the biggest day of your life is just another boring day at the office.

Our check-in clerk was an especially surly type. Still, I ended up liking her simply because she came up with one of the most creative ways of butchering a common colloquial expression that I'd ever heard: "Why don't you sit right here child, and we'll go ahead and send your wife to the delivery room. That way we can kill a bird with two of dem stones."

Of course, you could arrive at the hospital, get settled into a delivery room, and then be told by your doctor to go back home. This is more common than you think, and frankly, it sucks. All that emotion, that sudden rush of adrenaline—gone in a flash. You feel like you've been banished or exiled to "wait it out."

What's perhaps most amazing about this period is just how much women can accomplish. My friend Fern, who was desperate to sell her home (it had been on the market for nearly a year), actually agreed to give a tour to prospective buyers only an hour after being sent home from the hospital. Her husband tried to stop her, but it was too late. Some folks on a stroll in the neighborhood thought they were having an open house, so they asked if they could look around as well. With six people in tow and bone-crushing contractions, she began the tour. "Now . . . this . . . is . . . the . . . master . . . bedroom, hold it, wow, son-of-a-bitch that hurts. Oh sorry . . . okay, I'm back" The house was sold the following day.

Mother Teresa

ONCE you're settled in your hospital room, you'll meet your labor-and-delivery nurse. Don't underestimate the importance of this individual. No doubt you've been led to believe that the OB/GOD will be by your wife's side throughout the labor. Not so. The doctor will appear for periodic checks every couple of hours until your wife is ready to give birth, but for the most part he or she is missing in action. This not only came as a surprise to me, but it also pissed me off. After all, this whole birthing experience was costing me a fortune and I wanted my money's worth.

In contrast to your doctor's missing-in-action status, the labor-and-delivery nurse remains with you and your wife the entire time. So, if you are assigned Nurse Ratchet, request a replacement or discreetly ask when the next shift begins (read: when Nurse Ratchet is scheduled to go home). This is your comrade in arms, the one who will calm your wife when she is consumed with labor pains and begins to levitate. You and your wife must like her.

Riding the Wave

ONCE your wife is gingerly placed on the delivery bed or table, a fetal monitor will be strapped around her belly. This device, which is basically a pregnancy-style Richter scale, uses sound waves to measure the peaks and valleys of your wife's contractions. A separate computer-like screen displays the peaks and valleys in graph format.

When you see a contraction coming (you will often get the first glimpse at the monitor), this is the time to attempt those breathing exercises you and your wife so studiously mastered. Nada told me after the birth that she could tell when a bad contraction was coming just by the look on my face—like I just woke up naked in a crowded park. You should attempt to say and do things that may ease your wife's pain. Unfortunately, the only thing that really works will be more drugs.

The most important word in the English language at this point is *dilation*. Dilation of a woman's cervix is measured on a scale from one to ten. If your wife's cervix is dilated one or two centimeters, grab a good book because she's got a long way to go. Once her cervix is at ten centimeters, she's ready for liftoff.

I found the "science" of determining the extent to which a woman is dilated hardly exact. The doctor reaches up with his hand inside the opening, feels around a bit, and then announces "You're exactly X centimeters." How do they do that? With few exceptions, first-time births tend to go on for many hours. If dilation is especially slow, the doctor may give your wife a drug called Pitocin to help speed things up.

The Mother of All Shots: The Epidural

UPON arrival in your delivery suite, I would urge you to ask the nurse if you can get your wife an epidural. This is a shot of drugs to the spine that gradually takes away the immense pain experienced during labor. My friend Greta told me she made it to the hospital too far along into labor to receive this wonder drug (she was eight centimeters dilated, which is usually the cut-off point). During one heavy contraction, she attempted

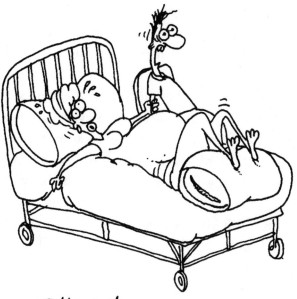

It's not uncommon for
both partners to become dilated
at the same time.

to bite the nurse who told her she would have to do without. You should take no chances that your wife will miss the boat.

Of course, this information about the epidural is completely useless if you and your wife have decided to go drug-free. No problem with this, but just be prepared if she finds the pain too severe to handle and begins to sound like a heroin addict: "Get me some drugs, *bastard*!" My holistic friend Steve tried to dissuade his wife from using drugs, even after she complained of unbearable pain. "Remember, we swore to keep the birth drug-free for the sake of the baby," he kept reminding her. "*I said*, get me an epidural, *idiot*!" she responded. If your wife is crying out in agony for an epidural, do her, and yourself, a favor: Call for the anesthesiologist.

The Only Day She'll Pray to Be Constipated

I BET one of your wife's biggest fears about the birth is the possibility of passing more than just the baby on the table. One guy I know swears his wife inquired about having her butt sewn shut for the delivery just to avoid the possibility.

If your wife is sweating about this common occurrence, you can assure her that with all that's going on down there, no one will really notice. Some women worry that their husbands will feel differently about them sexually if *it* happens. Come on, we're guys, we name our sex organ so that it won't be a stranger making 90 percent of our decisions. The real question is whether our spouse will still want to have sex with us.

You Have to Go Through Hell Before You Get to Heaven

A FEW months before our "big day" I heard a segment on National Public Radio that featured several pediatricians debating the merits of husbands in the delivery room. They cited statistics indicating that in the United States, eight out of ten men are present during the birth, and they argued that in some cases, women—and doctors—are better off going it alone with the dads sitting it out in a waiting room. This is particularly true, they said, for men who have difficulty coping with the sight of blood.

They interviewed a new dad who described his

wife's vaginal birth as the "Saturday Night Massacre." He hated the sight of blood, but he wanted to be supportive during the delivery. He and his wife therefore came to an agreement they called the "above-the-elbow rule." As long as he remained that high up, he was certain he could stay on his feet the entire time. The doctor on call when his wife was ready to deliver had little sympathy for this dad's discomfort. "Either get down here and help, or get out of the room," he said. Not wanting to disappoint his wife or appear like a wimp in front of the doctor, the guy headed south. "I fought the good fight," he said, "but it was a bit too much for me to handle. I was on the floor sucking tile in a matter of minutes."

If you start feeling a little queasy during the birth, know that you are not alone. Try the above-the-elbow rule. Most doctors will understand—and will be much happier to have only one patient at a time.

If it becomes necessary for your wife to go the alternate route, the infamous C-section, don't panic. And don't be surprised, when the doctor announces this decision, if your wife gives you a look of disappointment, followed by another of sheer terror—something akin to the look of a death-row inmate headed for the electric chair. Some women believe they've failed the first test of motherhood by not delivering the baby the "natural" way. Other women who have had a previous C-section may actually prefer it over a vaginal delivery because there is no pain involved during the procedure. However, the healing process tends to be much longer and more painful after a Cesarean delivery.

The medical team performing the surgery has been through the C-section drill a zillion times. As such, they may appear a bit too lax about the whole affair for your comfort. Several couples told me that their surgeons engaged in casual chatter—about their kids, the movies, sports—while performing the surgery. If this happens to you, the temptation to interrupt may be overwhelming: "Uh, now I may be out of line here, but with my wife's guts hanging out and all, do you think maybe you can *shut up* till the operation's over? Just a suggestion."

True story. A friend who worked in a pizza place during college. One day, a young guy came into the store, viewed the various pizzas on display, and then ordered "a slice of Cesarean with pepperoni."

If your wife is on target for a vaginal delivery, the doctor will at some point make the critical announcement: "It's time to push!" If an epidural has been administered, the dosage will be dropped so she can use her strength to help get the baby out. Either way, she'll feel every scintilla of pain in the now near-constant, volcanic-like contractions. It is at this point that she may begin throwing verbal spears around the room. Get ready to duck.

The birthing room suddenly transforms from common hotel lodging into the set of *ER*. (A special anteroom may be prepared to clean the baby upon its arrival.) The doctor gets in position. (I kept waiting for him to say, "Hey batter, batter," his crouch reminded me of a baseball catcher waiting for a pitch.) When your baby begins to emerge, take a snap-shot in your mind. This is the moment you will never want to forget. I can still see—and hear—it vividly.

"Oh my god," I called out. "Here comes the head. But . . . but . . . she's not breathing! Dr. Newman, I think she's dead!"

He calmly informed me that the baby was still attached to the umbilical cord, which had been feeding oxygen into her lungs for the past nine months.

"I knew that, I was just making sure." I knew at that moment that I'd lost every shred of credibility with him, not that I had much to begin with. But what about the shape of my angel's head? My wife had just given birth to Veldar, the conehead. "Dr. Newman, her head, well, I mean, it's pointy. It kind of looks like a conehead." How would I explain to my parents that their first and only grandchild looked like a character from Saturday Night Live?

"That's normal," the doctor reassured me, probably wondering why he ever agreed to allow me in the room in the first place. "Babies' skulls are so soft at birth that they often exit the birth canal slightly misshapen. Your baby's head will round out in a couple of days.

"You sure about that?"

"Yes, I'm sure."

"Thank god."

Once the baby's body fully emerges and the doctor clamps the umbilical cord, you may be asked to cut the cord. Some men feel honored, others feel sick to the stomach, and still others fear hurting the baby. Your choice. The baby is then placed on the mother's chest for warmth or taken to an anteroom for an initial cleanup. Now this is where I thought things ended. What I hadn't truly appreciated is that women have to give birth to a second child, named "Placenta." (If she has a C-Section, this mass of bodily gook, which looks like a big hunk of liver, is taken out for her before she is sewn back up.) This requires even more pushing. The placenta will be followed by other indescribable matter, and a final check by the doctor to make sure nothing is left in there that may cause infection.

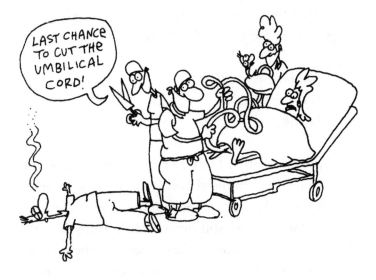

The Third Trimester: (7 Months to Delivery)

Then, as if to take away any joy your wife may be feeling at this moment, out come needle and thread. During a vaginal delivery, either the doctor performed an episiotomy (making a slit in her stretching skin to ease the passage of the baby) or the skin tore on its own. In either case, it's time for doc to play Betsy Ross—and for your wife to wonder "Will this hell ever end?" It was at this moment when Nada, who had survived nearly fifteen hours of intense labor, turned to me and said, "God hates women."

Where's My Reward?

YOUR wife has just been through hell and back. Don't be surprised if she's expecting a significant token of your appreciation for her bravery and the miracle of having produced your first born. "Women want a medal for what they have to do with their bodies. And that medal should be made of gold," one woman advised me. My friend Sarah told me she wanted one carat weight for every centimeter she was dilated.

If you decide to buy your wife a gift, you may be tempted to come up with something creative, perhaps related to the birthing experience. Be careful. My friend Philip gave his wife a pair of thick thermal socks, which he thought was a perfect gift because she had complained of cold feet throughout her pregnancy. He was a bit surprised by her reaction. "My crotch has just been spread from New York to L.A. and all I get is socks. Go to hell!" She didn't talk to him for several hours.

The Fun Begins!

ONCE your wife is settled into a maternity room, your baby will be brought to the room. Unless you've had some past experience with infants, you'll probably be thinking, "You're not going to leave her with us alone, are you?" I was tempted to say, "If you care about the health of this baby, if this is a reputable medical institution, you will *not* leave her in here with us!" Your wife may feel more confident about handling the baby than you do, but she'll be so wiped out that you'll wonder if she'll ever have the strength to get out of bed.

It's an Asian custom to say a newborn is ugly, regardless of its actual appearance, in order to prevent jealous spirits from attacking the baby with illness. Since most newborns *are* ugly, you'll probably have little trouble observing this custom. Babies delivered by Cesarean are a notable exception to this rule, but newborns delivered vaginally often look like a cross between a wilted China doll and a bewildered Telly Savalas. Some newborns will make you wonder whether Henny Youngman was really joking when he said he was such an ugly baby that the doctor slapped his mother.

Because so few babies are attractive right from the start, it's always fun to see how your parents and other visitors react to seeing your kid for the first time. Only your closest friends will tell you the truth: "Man, what's the deal with the conehead?" is how my friend Dave reacted after seeing Logan for the first time.

Nothing is more exciting or gratifying than getting your new baby into the car for the trip home from the hospital. You know you've just crossed the threshold between having a baby and starting a new life and family with one. The first few days at home can be extraordinarily difficult and exhausting. Your wife will be completely exhausted and extremely sore, and she'll have only limited mobility. She'll also have enough milk in her breasts to feed a small army, caus-ing her breasts to swell with soreness and in size—big enough to rest her chin on. You will feel inept at diaper changing at first, and think that your crying infant is saying "Get me somebody who knows what they're doing or I'll keep screaming." Bathing, cleaning, dressing, and doing just about everything else with the baby will all seem like a huge challenge. Don't expect more than two hours of sleep at one time. Do expect huge bags under your eyes. They signal your entrance into the world's most exclusive club: fatherhood.

A close friend's wife suffered from a crippling case of constipation after she gave birth to twins. She called Nada one Saturday afternoon a week after the birth pleading for her to fetch an enema since her husband needed to stay home to watch the babies. I reluctantly volunteered to go. If you've ever purchased an enema, maybe you can relate. Buying an enema is like buying a condom for the first time, only worse. Of course, the drugstore I went to had them hidden. I was forced to ask the clerk, who had a voice like a megaphone, "YOU LOOKIN' FOR AN ENEMA!!!? AISLE 7." Now that the whole store knew, I grabbed two (99 cents each, what a bargain). "How much do I owe you?" my friend asked. "It's on me," I said. "I always wanted to treat a friend to an enema."

Things No One Tells You About the Post-Delivery Experience

1. Your wife will leave the hospital looking pregnant and remain that way for several weeks. Even with newborn in tow, people will ask her, "So, when are you due?" This is a surefire way to piss her off.

2. You'll need a second car or flatbed truck to bring home the gifts you receive at the hospital. You'll love all the flowers and food, but where the hell do you put them all?

3. You'll lose count of the number of strangers who have seen your wife naked. Okay, it's medical and all. Still, you'll swear there were guys coming in and out of the room just to catch a peek.

4. You'll discover that the official food of new fathers is cereal. You may get a home-cooked meal once in a while, but it ain't going to be from your home.

Slice and Dice

To cut or not to cut? That's a profound question, especially for an interfaith couple with a baby boy. Nada, who is Catholic, was all for circumcision, but not in the fashion common to my side of the family—at a celebration called a *bris*. I'm not sure how the founding fathers of Judaism came up with this practice, but a bris is essentially a party centered on watching a newborn boy get cut by a guy called a *mohel*, which means "penis slicer" in Yiddish. How do people get into this profession? "Mommy, when I grow up, I want to be a mohel." Has that ever happened? Anyway, Nada was not enamored of the idea of a traditional bris. "If my kid's gonna get his dick cut," she said, "I don't want it to happen in front of an audience stuffing their faces with bagels and lox."

Final Words

WRITING this book has been much like reliving the pregnancy experience, except it's been a lot more fun. The project generated plenty of laughs among myself, my wife, and our friends as we reviewed the trials and tribulations of couples going through a pregnancy. I hope you had a few laughs, too, and maybe even learned something useful along the way.

In my view, the most shocking thing about pregnancy is just how fast women bounce back both physically and mentally after the baby is born. Or, perhaps even more amazing is their ability to put all the pain and misery of labor and delivery behind them. Before you know it, your wife will be talking about having another baby. At least you'll *really* know what to expect.

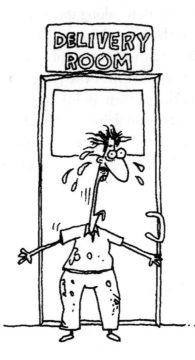

One of the best things to come out of being present during the birth is that changing a diaper (something you've dreaded from the start) will now be a piece of cake.

Epilogue

NADA AND I were in Los Angeles on our first vacation since the baby was born. We were a block from the famous Rodeo Drive in Beverly Hills. I was looking out the window of our rented Ford Taurus (they were all out of minivans) thinking how great life really is with a baby. Now six months old, Logan was just beginning to develop a personality all her own. She was in the backseat playing with her favorite new toy—a Fisher Price radio—and singing "la la la la." I looked in the rearview mirror. *My wife and my baby on Rodeo Drive.* I am one cool guy . . . but wait. The radio fell out of Logan's hand onto her nose. She launched into a silent scream.

"Ian, she looks pretty upset," Nada said. "I think she's going to throw up."

"Oh, she's fine," I responded, as if I knew what I was talking about.

Two seconds later Linda Blair was in the backseat acting out a scene from *The Exorcist.* Logan and Nada and their expensive Rodeo Drive outfits were all covered in you-know-what. We were an hour's drive from our hotel.

After cleaning up as best we could, we decided we needed to get some clean clothes for Logan. Nada was adamant that we continue on, as she was—determined to show those "Beverly Hills snobs" that she could stand tall with puke stains all over her shirt. I admired her self-confidence, but wondered if the odor would be too much to take. We stripped the baby down, parked the car, and began our mission.

"Excuse me. But would you happen to know where we could find a Baby Gap?" I asked a saleswoman at a chic clothing store where socks cost $30 a pair. She looked like an emaciated Cindy Crawford, with a pierced—tongue? Man, that's gotta hurt.

"Like, that ith thso cool," she responded with a soft lisp, probably caused by the tongue ring. "I mean, you have the baby in justht a diaper. Almothst naked. Thso

free. Thso relaxed. I admire you two thso much." Is she
for real? "And those earrings." We had Logan's ears
pierced at three months. "He looks thso cute with them."
Now I knew she was on something or maybe all the hip
families in L.A. pierce their baby boys' ears. Fortunately,
she was lucid enough to direct us to the Baby Gap a few
blocks away.

Ahhh. Life with a baby. It's always expecting the unexpected. It's tough, amusing, and often exhausting. It's being bleary eyed and forever out of cash. And it's like nothing else in the world when you see your baby smile at you each day. You'll be smitten for life.

Acknowledgments

JUST ABOUT THE only one who didn't get sucked in to helping me with this book is my dog, Sandy. There are so many people to thank. To the pregnant couples at Montgomery Mall in Bethesda, Maryland, who agreed to talk with a total stranger about such a sensitive subject—what the hell were you thinking? To my friends who grudgingly read and reread draft after draft: Lionel Johnson, Gary Orseck, Michael Madonna, and so many others—don't even think about touching my royalties. As my daughter, who has yet to learn how to share would say "they're MINE." Special thanks go to my agent, Kevin Lang at the Bedford Book Works, who kept the faith that indeed these boys would swim, to Lorna Dolley Eby at Prima Publishing for proving him right, to my parents for their constant encouragement and to Steve Skelton for the hilarious and irreverent illustrations. And finally, to my wife, Nada, who started scouting out the jewelry counters at Neiman Marcus as soon as the book was purchased. She's convinced it will be a bestseller. Given the prices at Neiman's, please don't let her down.

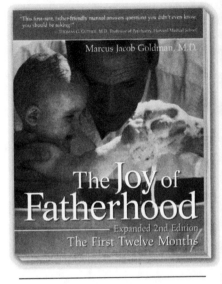

About the Author

New father Ian Davis is a lobbyist in Washington, D.C., for a Fortune 500 company. If you have any hilarious pregnancy-related stories, please send them to me at:

4408 Leland Street
Chevy Chase, MD 20815